We dedicate this book to all the children, and youth, along with their families and loved ones, who are courageoulsy battling Leukemia, and all the amazing providers who care for them.

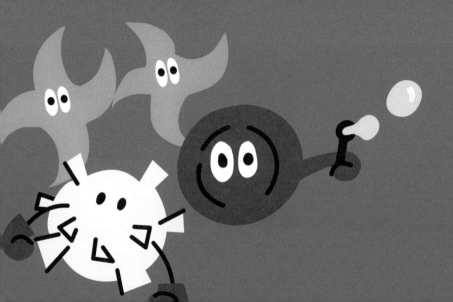

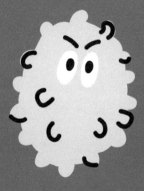

For information please contact author at hello@childcorefamilysupport.com

ISBN: 9798396671195

The information in this book is designed to be used as a starting point to educate a child
on the topic of a bone marrow transplant and not in lieu of supports or consults
from Certified Child Life Specialist, or other medical professionals.

For more information about Child Life Specialists
and how they can help, go to childcorefamilysupport.com.

Written + Illustrated by Adrienne O'Connor, MS, CCLS
Written by Caitlin McNamara, MS, CCLS, CIMI

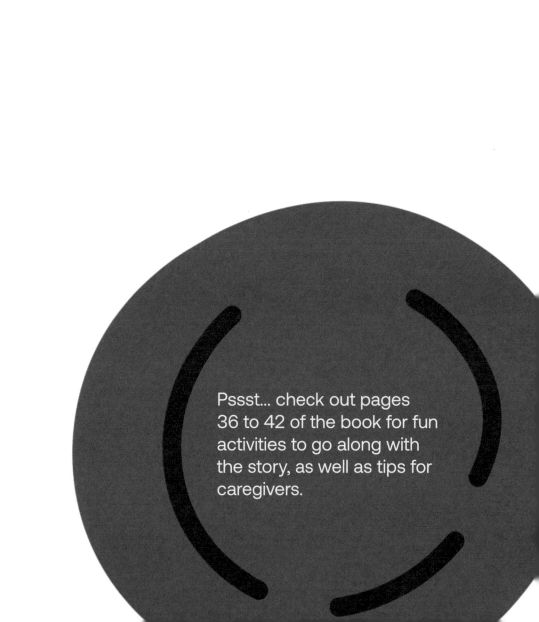

Pssst... check out pages 36 to 42 of the book for fun activities to go along with the story, as well as tips for caregivers.

Hi Friends!
Have you ever heard the word

Leukemia?
(Lou-kee-mee-uh)

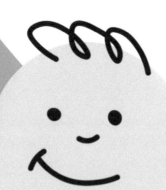

Leukemia is something that happens inside the body, it is when someone's blood gets sick.

Before I share more about leukemia, it can be helpful to understand how the inside of the body works.

Let me share what I have learned with you.

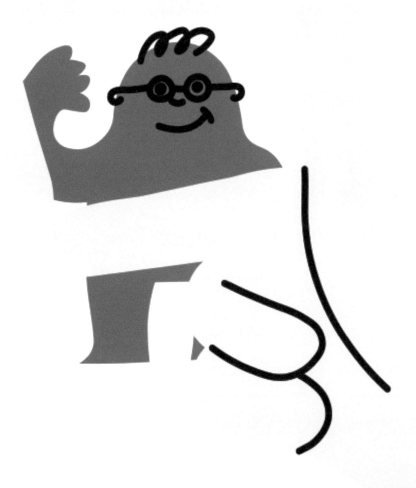

The inside of our bodies are made up of different systems that all work together.

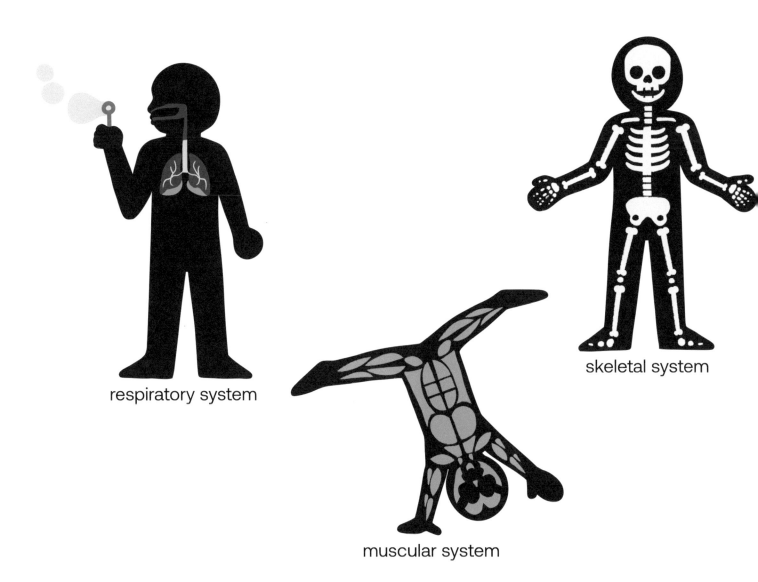

respiratory system

muscular system

skeletal system

All of these systems have different jobs,

and they work together so we can do things like run, play, eat, breathe, and use our imagination.

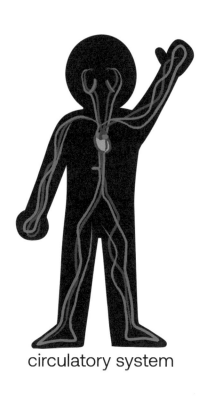

circulatory system

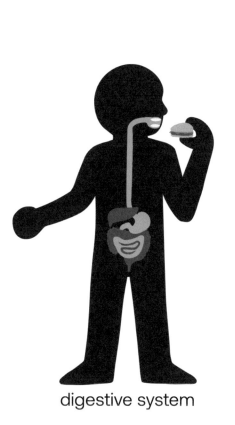

digestive system

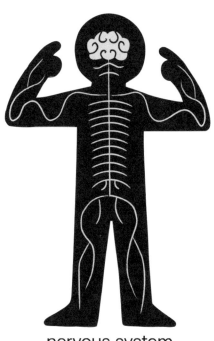

nervous system

Now, let's take a closer look at the circulatory system, or the blood system.

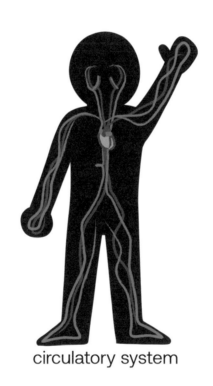

circulatory system

The blood system is made up of tunnels called veins and arteries.

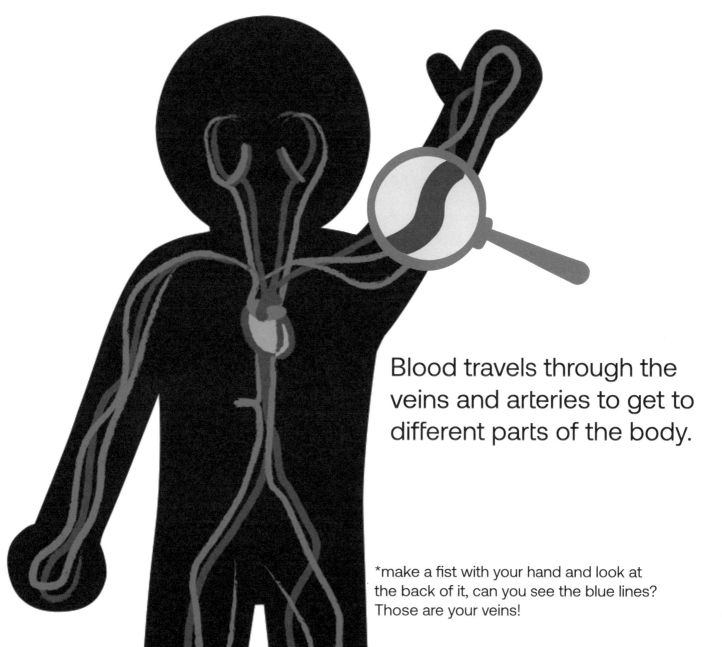

Blood travels through the veins and arteries to get to different parts of the body.

*make a fist with your hand and look at the back of it, can you see the blue lines? Those are your veins!

9

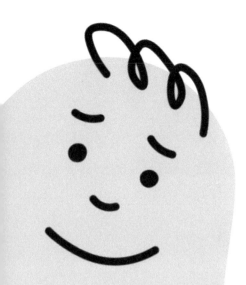

Did you know that blood has a very important job?

Blood carries things called CELLS to different parts of our body. Each type of cell has a different way it helps to keep our body healthy.

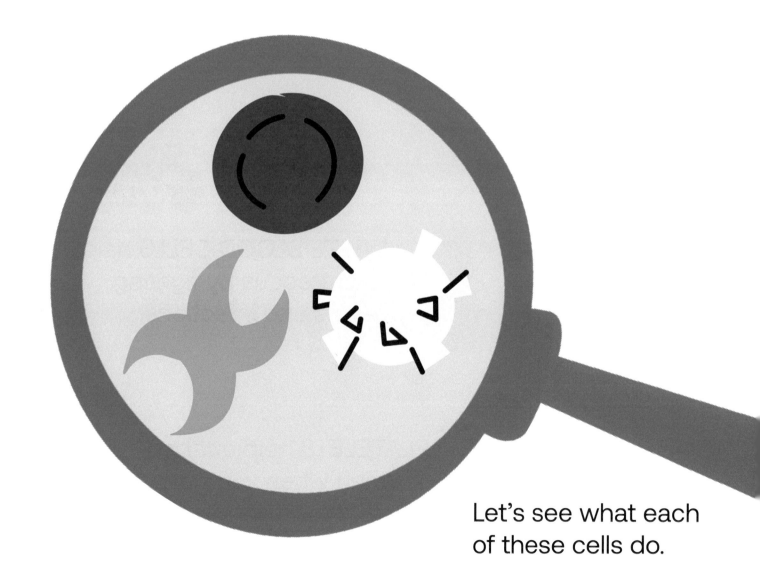

Let's see what each of these cells do.

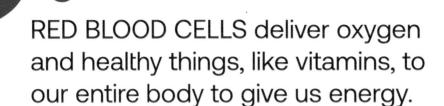

RED BLOOD CELLS deliver oxygen and healthy things, like vitamins, to our entire body to give us energy.

WHITE BLOOD CELLS help to protect us by fighting germs and infections.

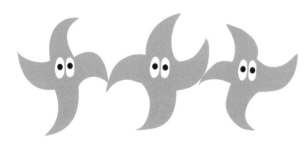

PLATELETS help our body heal. Think of when when you get a cut or a bruise, your platelets clump together to form a seal, or scab, to stop the bleeding.

These cells travel around in the liquid part of the blood called PLASMA.

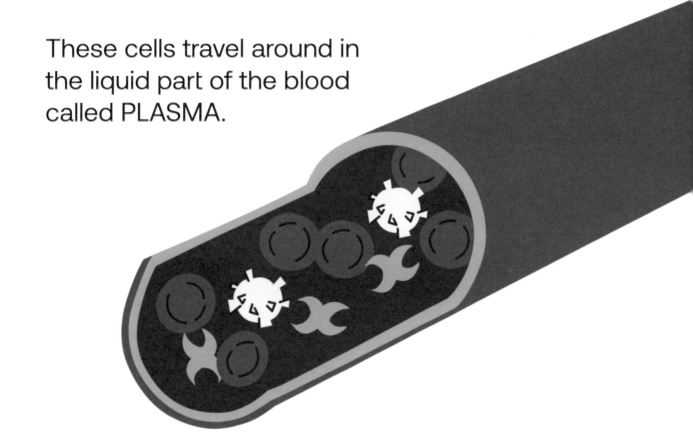

Ok, now that we've learned more about how the inside of the body works, I want to share with you what I learned about leukemia.

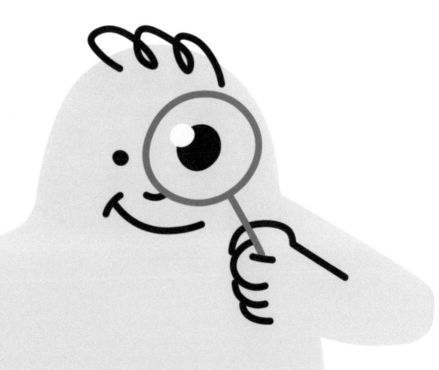

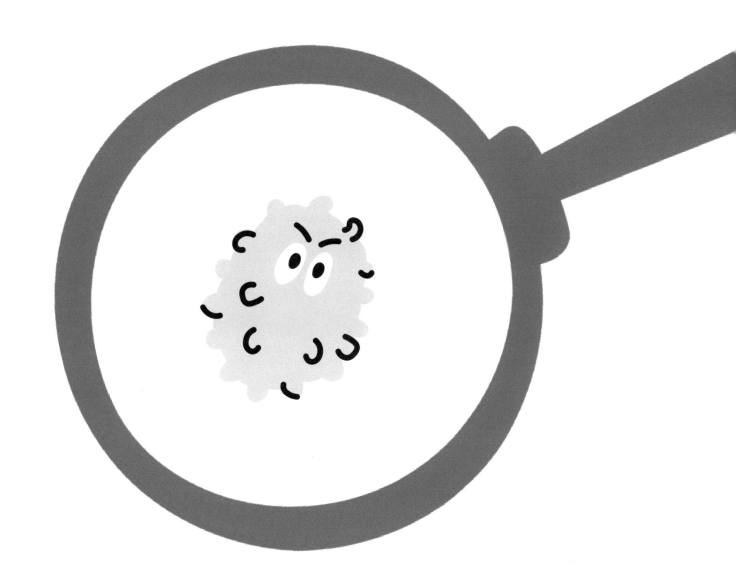

Leukemia is when someone has another type of cell in their blood, called a LEUKEMIA CELL or a BLAST CELL.

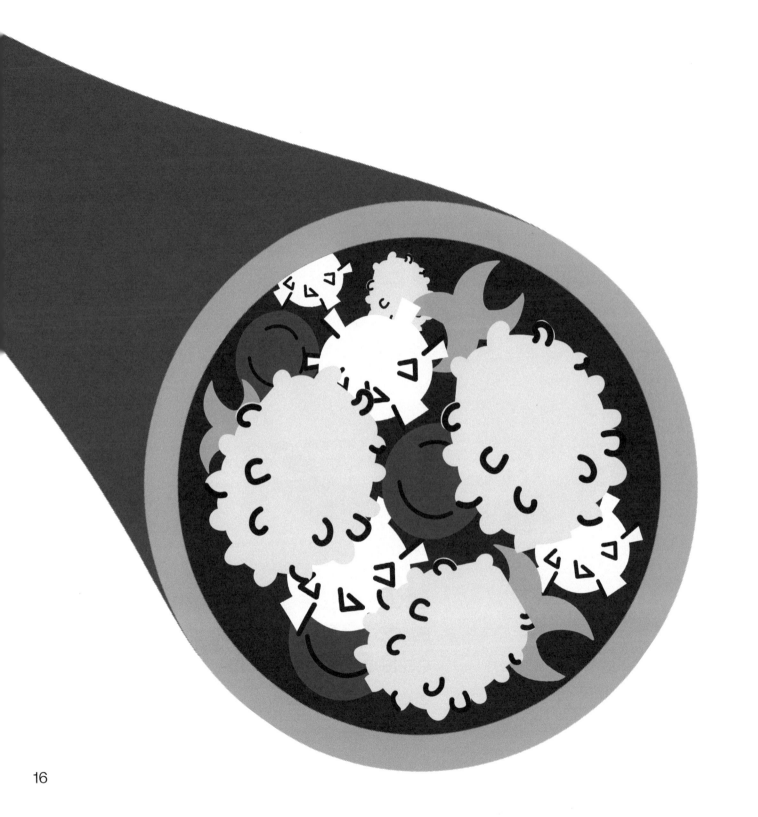

The blast cells block the tunnels (veins/arteries) and make it hard for the red blood cells, white blood cells, and platelets to travel through the body and do their jobs.

Kind of like a traffic jam.

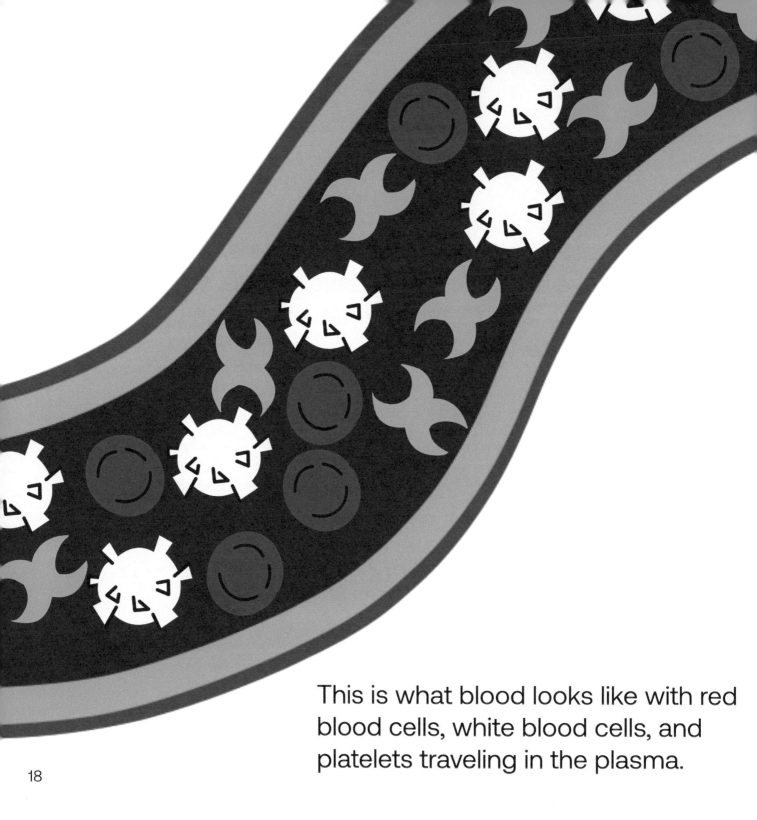

This is what blood looks like with red blood cells, white blood cells, and platelets traveling in the plasma.

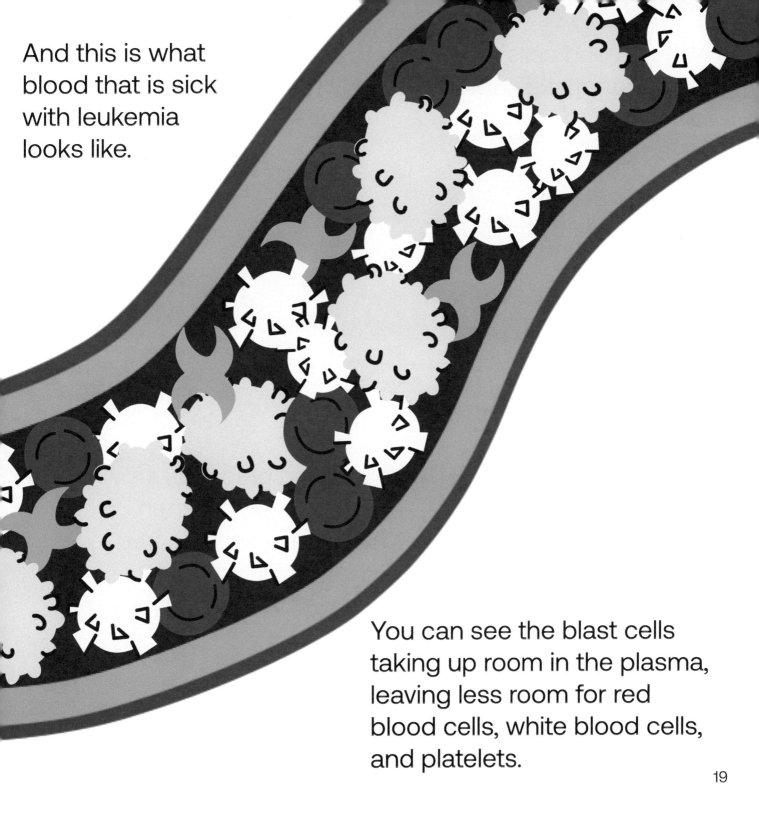

And this is what blood that is sick with leukemia looks like.

You can see the blast cells taking up room in the plasma, leaving less room for red blood cells, white blood cells, and platelets.

19

When blood cells are unable to do their job, it can make someone's body feel different...

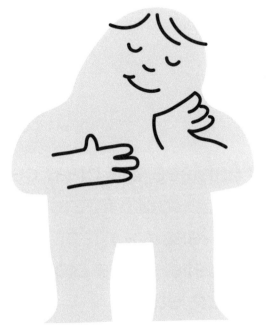

If their red blood cells can't do their job, then their body may feel tired.

If their white blood cells can't do their job, then their body may not be able to fight off germs, and they may feel sick.

If their platelets can't do their job, then their body may take a long time to heal from a cut or a bruise.

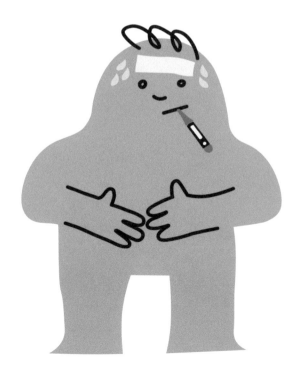

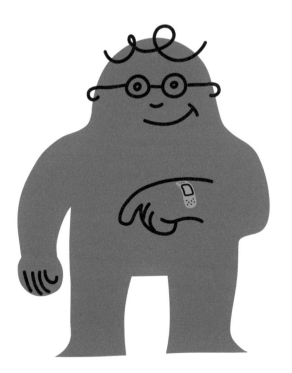

Leukemia is a different kind of
sick than when you have a cold
or the flu.

It is not contagious, meaning you can't
get leukemia by being near someone
who has it.

Doctors do not know why some people get leukemia and some people do not.

It is not because of something someone did or thought. Leukemia is no one's fault.

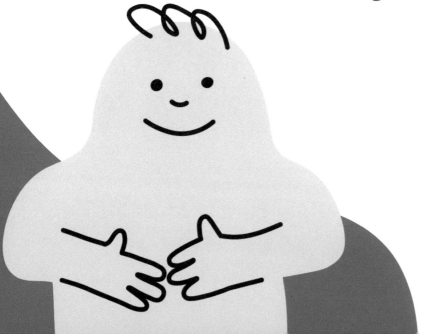

23

After I learned about leukemia, my next question was: how does someone get rid of the leukemia cells and help their body feel better?

Here is what I learned...

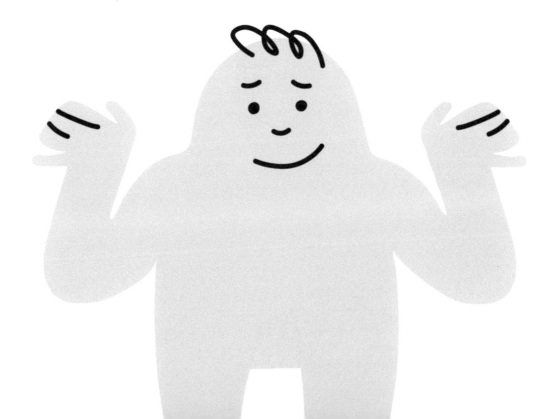

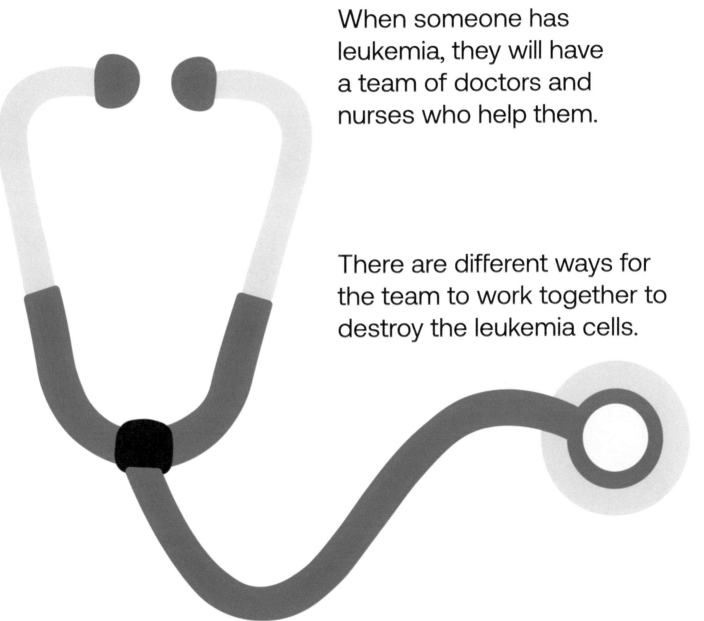

When someone has leukemia, they will have a team of doctors and nurses who help them.

There are different ways for the team to work together to destroy the leukemia cells.

The team might use RADIATION to help someone get rid of leukemia cells.

Radiation comes from a machine. The machine sends a powerful, invisible beam to the leukemia cells to destroy them.

Invisible means that the person can't see or feel the beams.

Like a superhero who aims their x-ray vision at bad guys, radiation is aimed directly at blast cells.

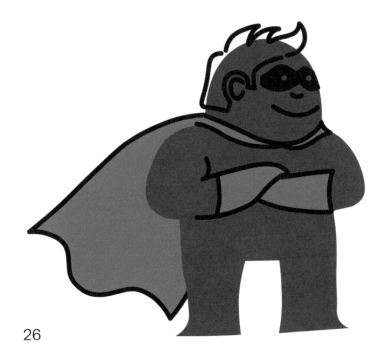

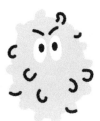

A second way the team can help someone get rid of leukemia cells is giving them a medicine called CHEMOTHERAPY (or chemo).

Which I learned is a strong medicine that helps to get rid of blast cells....

... kind of like an eraser!

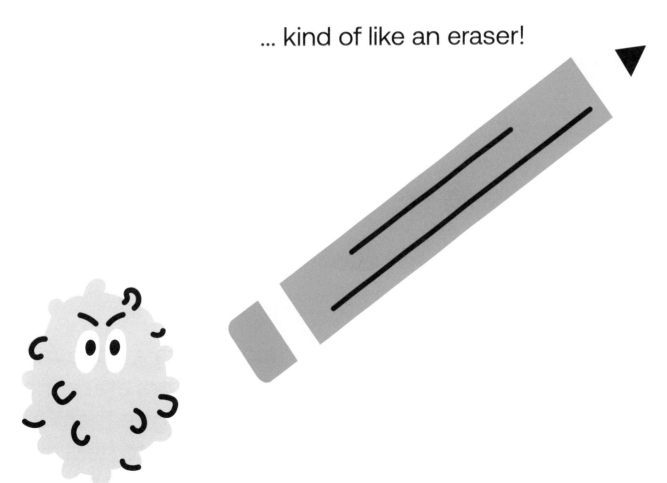

A third way to help someone get rid of leukemia cells is with a BONE MARROW TRANSPLANT.

Inside of the bones there is a blood making factory called BONE MARROW, where all of the blood cells are made.

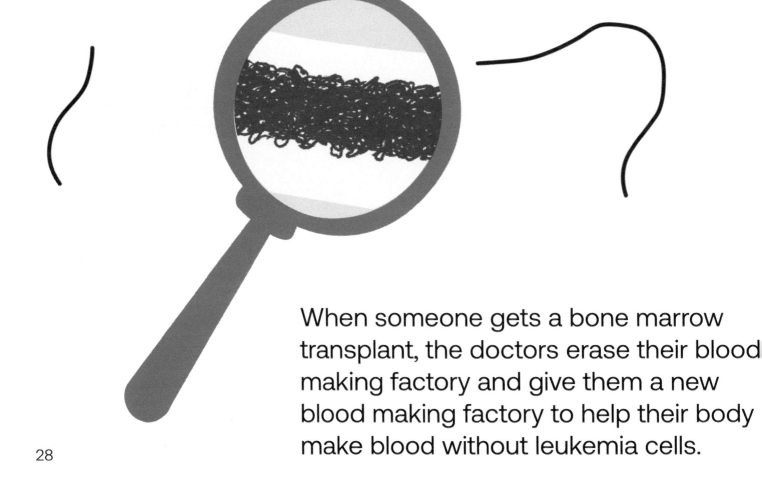

When someone gets a bone marrow transplant, the doctors erase their blood making factory and give them a new blood making factory to help their body make blood without leukemia cells.

Kind of like when someone plants a new garden. They get rid of the dirt and weeds first to make room for healthy soil and new flowers to grow.

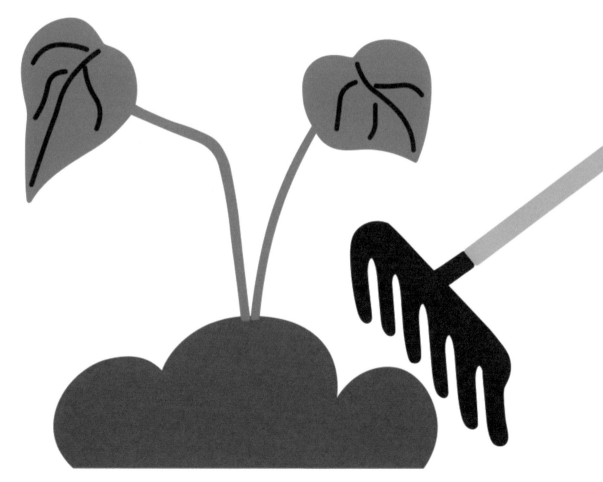

When someone is getting help for leukemia,
their body might look and feel different.

They might
lose their hair.

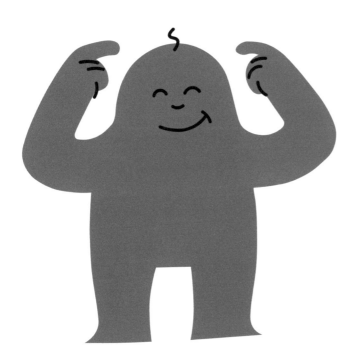

They might
feel tired.

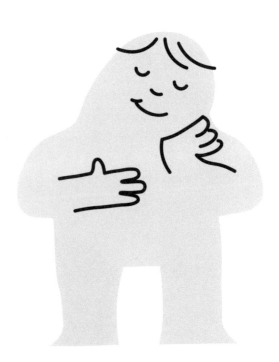

But there are ways doctors, nurses, and loved ones can help them feel better.

And when they no longer need help from their team because all the blast cells are destoryed, their body will start to look and feel more like themselves.

Their stomach might feel upset.

Their mouth and throat might feel yucky.

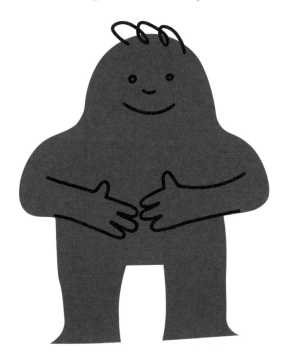

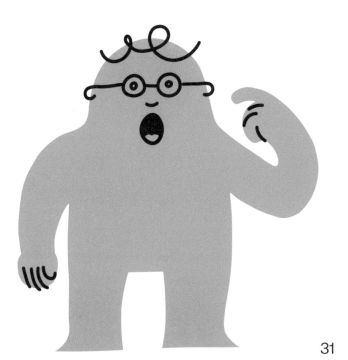

Wow, that was a lot of information. When I learn something new, it is helpful for me to talk to someone about what I learned, ask questions, and even go back and read things again.

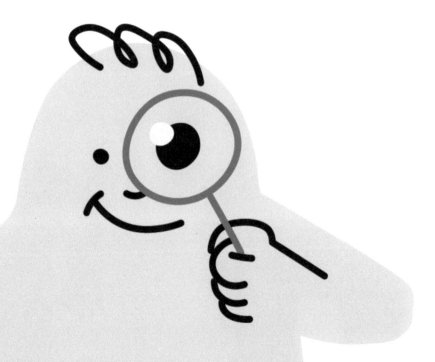

Thank you for letting me share what I learned with you, I wonder what I will learn about next!

Glossary

Cells:

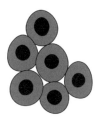

Cells are things that make up the body. They are so small you can't see them with your eyes, you need a microscope to see them. Every part of the body is made up of cells, both outside and inside. The body also makes and replaces cells all the time. There are lots of different types of cells and they all have unique jobs that work together to keep the body strong and healthy.

Circulatory system/blood system:

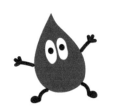

One of the body's systems that is made up of arteries and veins. Blood travels through these tunnels to get to different parts of the body.

Red Blood Cells:

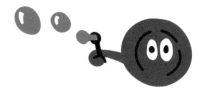

A type of cell that is found in the blood. Red blood cells carry nutrients, vitamins, and oxygen to the entire body, they also give the body energy to run, jump, and play.

White Blood Cells:

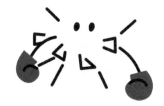

A type of cell that is found in the blood. White blood cells help fight off germs and help to keep the body healthy.

Platelets:

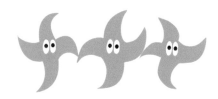

A type of cell that is found in the blood and helps the body heal. When someone's body gets hurt, platelets join together to form a seal to stop bleeding.

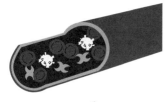

Plasma:

The liquid part of the blood that the cells travel in.

Leukemia cells/blast cells:

A type of cell that makes someone's blood sick because it should not be in the body and makes it hard for healthy cells to do their jobs.

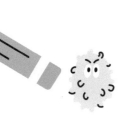

Chemotherapy:

Chemotherapy (chemo) is a strong medicine that gets rid of, or erases, blast cells.

Radiation:

A type of powerful, invisible beam that is used to help get rid of Leukemia cells. Invisible means the person can't see or even feel the beams.

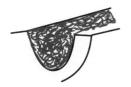

Bone Marrow:

The middle part of the bone where new blood cells are made, like a blood making factory.

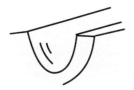

Bone Marrow Transplant:

A bone marrow transplant means getting new bone marrow to make healthy blood without blast cells.

Do you know someone who has leukemia?

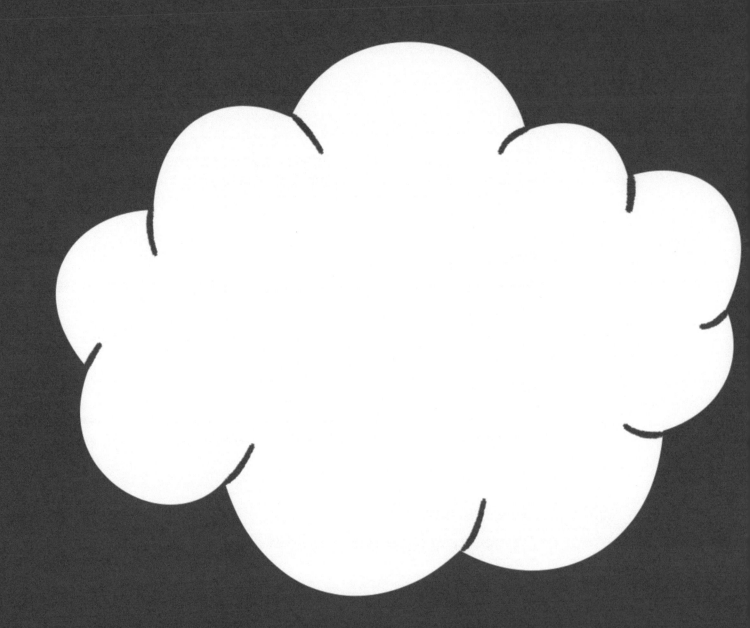

(here is where you can talk about someone
you know who is diagnosed with leukemia)

Think of some activities that children could
do in the hospital...

I wonder what questions you might have?
Or, if you have questions later, who would
you like to ask?

(draw a picture that could be hung up in the
hospital while you think about your questions)

Blood Cell Activity:

It is helpful for children to be introduced to new topics, especially abstract topics like leukemia, through hands-on activities. This can include, books, art projects, and/or through play.

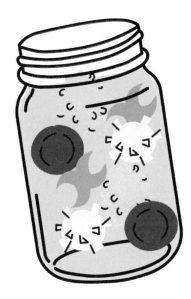

The Blood Cell Activity is a great activity to do in partnership with this book. It can aid in a child's learning and understanding of what blood looks like, what blood with leukemia looks like, and how leukemia cells disrupt the healthy blood cells functioning. At the end, the child will have a concrete representation they can physically hold and refer back too if needed.

This activity can be done for general learning purposes, for children diagnosied with leukemia, and/or for children who know someone who is impacted by leukemia.

For printable instructions:
Use your phone's camera to scan the QR code,
or visit www.childcorefamilysupport.com/blood-activity

FOR THE CAREGIVER:
Conversation Tips for Talking to Your Child About Leukemia

How to begin talking to your child about a leukemia diagnosis; whether it is someone they know or themselves with the diagnosis (pg. 36)

This book can serve as the entry point into a tough conversation. With this book, at any point – before, during, or after – you can assess if the child has ever heard these words and if so, what do they understand about them.

Children understand their world in concrete terms. Identifying physical symptoms they themselves, or someone they know, have experienced or witnessed, helps them make sense of information. For example, is someone feeling more tired or unable to engage in activities they enjoy? Do they bruise more easily? Have they had to spend time in the hospital receiving medicine?

If you are having a difficult time finding the right words to explain the "why," please contact us at hello@childcorefamilysupport.com to receive some 1:1 support on how to talk to your child about a diagnosis.

Brainstorming activities to do in a hospital setting (pg. 37)

When a child is in the hospital, it can be helpful to have activities to focus on. This helps provide an element of distraction, brings a sense of familiarity or comfort, and can even facilitate development and healing. Some examples are, color a picture to hang up in a hospital room, read books, watch movies, play games/cards, or do puzzles.

If your child or child's sibling is the one who is anticipated to be in the hospital for an extended period of time, include them in the experience of packing the hospital bag.

If it is a peer or family member that is anticipated to be in the hospital for an extended period of time, this could be a time to help the child think of a/an toy/item, or letter, or picture they could send along with them.

Checking-in about any questions your child may have or things they are curious about (pg. 38)

Children are curious about the world around them. It is important to create opportunities for children to have space and feel comfortable asking questions or sharing what they are wondering or worried about. This allows caregivers the chance to clarify any misconceptions (children have amazing imaginations), provide reassurance, and give information that is specific the individual child, thus, decreasing feelings of being overwhelmed with too much information.

You may be surprised at the things that are important to your child and thus, what their questions are. Some children need time to process information or they may need time to gather the courage to ask their questions. Therefore, check in with your child at various times following the book, this communicates to the child that the door is always open to talk to you and you are a safe space.

Scan the QR code to gain access to additional resources to help guide any adult through helping a child understand and cope with leukemia.

Scan with your phone's camera here!

Thank you to all of the Child Life Specialists
out there supporting children and their families!
We hope you hear it often,
you are doing amazing work!

Made in United States
Troutdale, OR
07/01/2024

20929320R00026